YOUR KNOWLEDGE HAS VALUE

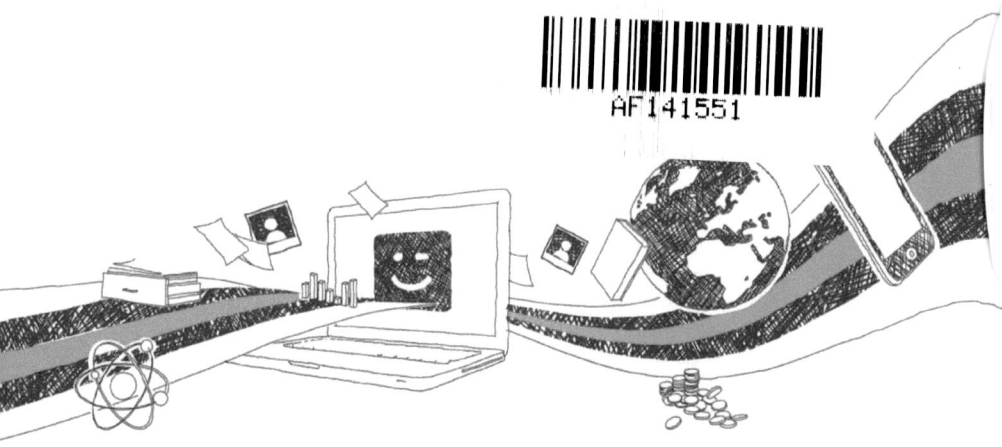
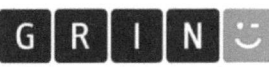

Bikal Dhungel

Challenges of Providing Primary Health Care

GRIN Publishing

Bibliographic information published by the German National Library:

The German National Library lists this publication in the National Bibliography;
detailed bibliographic data are available on the Internet at http://dnb.dnb.de .

Imprint:

Copyright © 2014 GRIN Verlag GmbH
Print and binding: Books on Demand GmbH, Norderstedt Germany
ISBN: 978-3-656-84153-1

This book at GRIN:

http://www.grin.com/en/e-book/283907/challenges-of-providing-primary-health-care

GRIN - Your knowledge has value

Since its foundation in 1998, GRIN has specialized in publishing academic texts by students, college teachers and other academics as e-book and printed book. The website www.grin.com is an ideal platform for presenting term papers, final papers, scientific essays, dissertations and specialist books.

Visit us on the internet:

http://www.grin.com/

http://www.facebook.com/grincom

http://www.twitter.com/grin_com

Challenges of Primary Healthcare for All and the Hindrance during and After a Violent Conflict: A Case Study of Nepal

By: Bikal Dhungel

Master of Science in Health Economics
College Of Life Sciences and Medicine
University of Aberdeen, United Kingdom 2

Abbreviations

ANMF: America Nepal Medical Foundation

GDP: Gross Domestic Product

GNI: Gross National Income

GNP: Gross National Product

GoN: Government of Nepal

ICRC: International Committee of Red Cross

IFAD: International Fund for Agricultural Development

LOC: Library of Congress

MDG: Millenium Development Goals

NGO: Non-governmental Organisations

NPR: Nepalese Rupees

OECD: Organisation of Economic Cooperation and Development

PHC: Primary Health Center

ROI: Return on Investment

SBA: Skilled Birth Attendance

SoE: State of Emergency

UNICEF: United Nations Children's Emergency Fund

USA: United States of America

USAID: United States Agency for International Development

VDC: Village Development Committee

WHO: World Health Organisation 3

Abstract

A challenge in providing Healthcare for all is a universal phenomenon. Especially developing countries lack the resources to fulfil this challenge. Additionally there are obstacles created both by the nature, due to complex geography which includes high mountains or hot desserts and by human themselves due to inefficient health policy, lack of proper manpower etc. Nepal is one of such countries that face serious challenge in delivering healthcare. It is not able to provide even a basic healthcare though it has signed every international treaties regarding health for example Alma-Ata Declaration. However, there has been some selective positive development. Still, multi-faceted challenges remain. Physical geography, its in-efficient bureaucracy, under-development, highly centralized health system and instable government contribute more to these challenges. A decade long civil war jeopardized the supply of healthcare taking the health system near to complete collapse in rural areas where majority of Nepalese reside. The burden of re-building is immense and fulfilling the Millennium Development Goals is unlikely. Given the direct and indirect cost incurred by a violent civil war like in Nepal, it turns to be a real tragedy where the most vulnerable are hit hard. Consequences of not being able to get proper care especially during and after childbirth for women and the lack of treatment facilities for those who need the most like TB patients, HIV positives, and millions of others who suffer from prevalent diseases like Malaria, Pneumonia, Measles etc. are immeasurable. It gives us a lesson that especially in such a poor setting, avoiding the conflict at any cost is vital. Moreover, there should be laws and treaties that ensure the security of health personnel who choose to save lives of others even in dangerous circumstances. It should be generally accepted that health is wealth and healthy citizens means a high potential of further economic development. 4

CONTENTS

1) Introduction: The WHO Constitution enshrines the highest attainable standard of health as a fundamental right of every human being. The right to health includes access to timely, acceptable and affordable healthcare of appropriate quality (WHO, 2013). However, billions of people especially in developing countries lack any Healthcare services for various reasons. The vibrant challenges countries face hinders the supply of healthcare that is terribly necessary for rural population of poor countries. Consequently, the 'health capital' of poorest of the poors is dire. Most of the developing countries lie in tropical areas, between the tropic of cancer and the tropic of capricorn. These areas are prone to diseases. So, developing countries also face the lion's share of the burden of diseases and at the same time lack the financial means to tackle the problem.

Nepal is one example of such countries that face severe challenges related to healthcare. Its physical geography that consists of mostly hills and mountains and hot regions of Terai impose a serious challenge to provide healthcare. This problem is worsened by the given traditional values that are reluctant to adopt scientific ways of treatment. Additionally, there are issues like political instability, war, violence, gender discrimination, poverty etc. which add oil into the fire.

In this paper I will mainly focus on the challenges to provide primary healthcare for all in such setting like that in Nepal and how it is worsened by violent conflicts like war. After mentioning some basic health characteristics of Nepal, I will discuss further about the challenges we face due to the factors like geography, culture, governance and economic issues. In the following part, I will illustrate the main points about this essay namely the challenges during a violent conflict or civil war. In Nepal's case it was the maoist-led civil war. Finally, I will conclude the main points again.

2) Objective and Methods: Objective of this essay is to incorporate the challenges to provide healthcare in a poor country with the violent conflict to give a message of why such conflicts should be avoided with all means if we want to ensure the availability of healthcare for everybody in the present and in future which contributes to the overall economic development observing the case of Nepal. The objective is also to highlight the direct and indirect cost Nepal faces because of the civil war.

Literatures were searched and reviewed with the help of google, google scholar and medline. Additionally, an access to scientific papers was made available by the help of Kathmandu University medical school which allowed access to literatures about health that was related to Nepal and its system.

3) Overview of Nepalese Health Profile: Nepal is one of the least developed countries in the world that lies between two giants China and India. The following statistics have been provided by the World Health Organisation (WHO)

Total population (2012)	**27,474,000**
Gross National Income per capita (PPP international $, 2012)	**1,470**
Life expectancy at birth m/f (years, 2011)	**67/69**
Probability of dying under five (per 1000 live births, 2012)	**42**
Probability of dying between 15-60 years m/f (per 1000 population, 2011	**183/157**
Total expenditure on health per capita (Intl $, 2011)	**68**
Total expenditure on health as % of GDP (2011)	**5.4**

(Source: WHO, 2014)

With a GNP per capita of $1470 and a total expenditure on health per capita of $68, it shows that 4.6% of national income is spent on health. Comparing with developed countries with the help of following figure, it shows that in real numbers, the per capita expenditure is meagre but in terms of percentage of GDP, the number does not deviate much from those of richer countries.

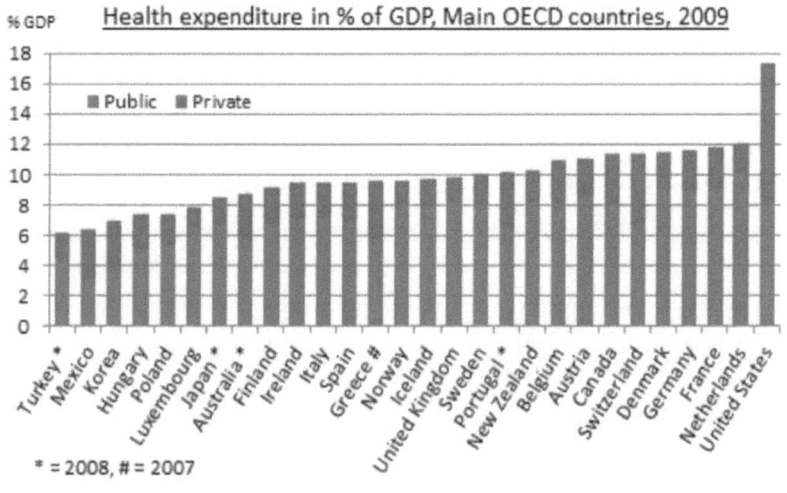

(Source: OECD statistics, 2013)

However, due to political instability and frequently changing government, healthcare expenditure in total as well as per capita also changes with it. The following two figures shows the expenditure related to GDP and Per Capita. From this, we can conclude that health spending is very inconsistent and imbalanced.

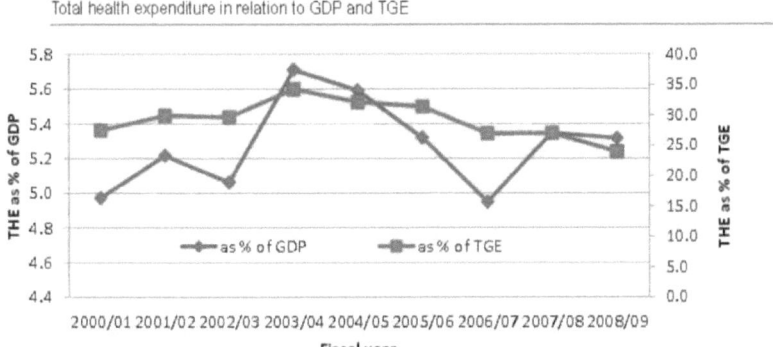

(Source: OECD Statistics, 2014)

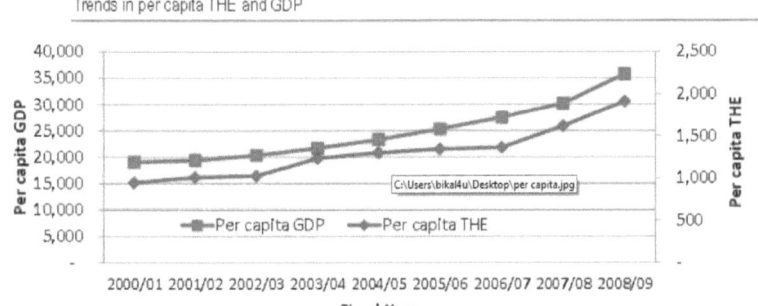

(Source: OECD Statistics, 2014)

4) Economics of Health Sector: There are 20 medical colleges in Nepal. Most of them are private. These 20 colleges can accommodate roughly 2000 students per year. However, roughly 8000 students want to study medicine. Those who cannot make the entry examination either opt to study something else or go to foreign countries mainly to China, India, Bangladesh, Pakistan and Germany (because of its free education). Average fee for the entire medical education is around 4.2 million NPR (~ 35,000£) (Dixit, 2008)

There are 0.24 physicians per 1000 individuals and estimated 1.9 hospital beds per 100,000 people

Regarding Nurses, there are 117 Nursing campuses till date. There are 40,000 nurses currently employed which includes roughly 1000 foreign nurses (Marahatta,Dixit,2008) who came to Nepal to do volunteering through charities or other international cooperation programs.

Additionally, following relevant data is available from the Ministry of Health (2014):
⬚

- Top ten diseases accounting for morbidity:

Pyrexia of unknown origin:	3.7
Headache:	3.7
Gastritis (APD)	3.6
ARI (Lower Respiratory Infection)	3.6
Upper Respiratory Tract Infection	3.4
Intestinal Worm	3.2
Amoebic Dysentery	2.2
Falls/Injuries	2

(Source: Nepalese Ministry of Health, 2014)

- Maternal Health

Antenatal Care from Skilled Birth Attendants (SBA)	58.3%
Percentage of births protected against neonatal tetanus	81.5%
Delivery at home	63.1%
Delivery at health facility	35.3%

(Source: Nepalese Ministry of Health, 2014)

- Child Health   (Immunization)

BCG	97
DPT 3	91.4
Polio 3	92.1
Measles	88
None	2.9

(Source: Nepalese Ministry of Health, 2014)

- Health Facilities under Ministry of Health and Population

Hospitals (central, regional, sub-regional, zonal and district)	86
Primary Health Center (PHC)	205
Health Post	822
Sub-Health Post	2987
Health Volunteers	48897

(Source: Nepalese Ministry of Health, 2014)

5) Challenges of Providing Primary Healthcare

5.1) Physical Geography:

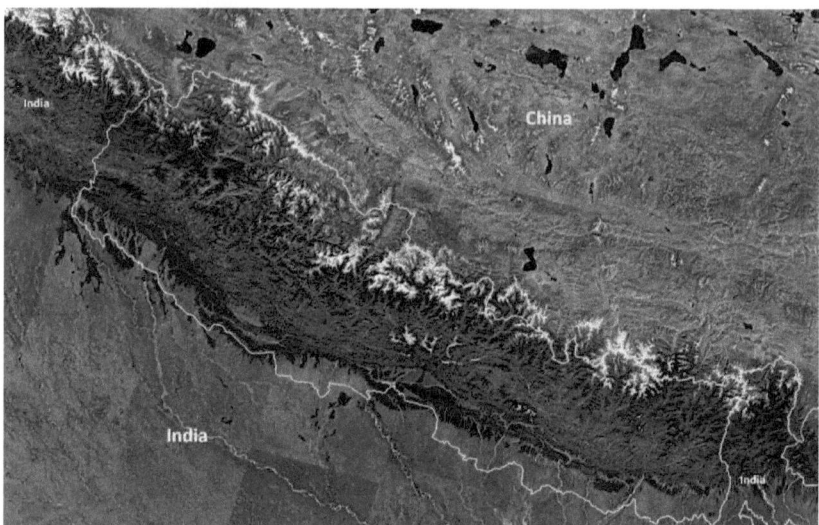

Source: Cut from Google Maps

The map of Nepal reveals that it is mainly hills and mountains. 80% of the total population lives in rural areas (IFAD, 2013) which possess a threat to accessibility. Lack of physical infrastructures like roads and bridges is especially a problem is rural areas. Medical supplies are difficult to transport in such condition hence porters are used to carry out weeks long perilous journeys to reach the particular areas. On the way, medicines are prone to get damaged due to severe weather conditions or there is a risk that porters themselves do not survive the journey.

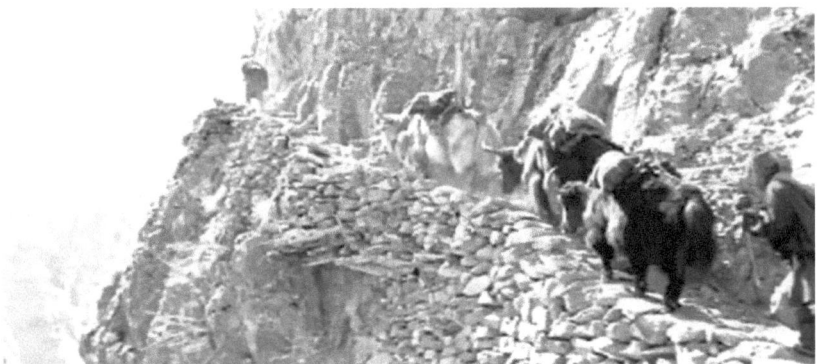

Source: Cut from the Film Caravan, 2001 (Goods are being transported with the help of Yaks)

5.2) Highly Centralized Health System: Most hospitals (90%) are located in urban areas (LOC, 2005) where only 20% of total population reside. Rural areas with its 80% share of total population are left with severe scarcity of health professionals mainly doctors and nurses. There is one hospital or health center in most of the districts but due to a long journey people have to undertake, they opt for alternative way of treatment which is some religious or traditional practice. Since most of the health centers and hospitals are understaffed and over-crowded because of the number of people they should treat, rural inhabitants have less incentive to start the journey.

Rural dwellers also require more care due to their lifestyles for example climbing trees for chopping woods for domestic fires or gathering leaves as cattle fodder it is not surprising that injuries as a result of falls are quite common. Walking along mountain trials in the dark can be cause of falls leading to broken bones or even death (LOC, 2005)

Since it is expensive to get medical education, only the children of elite families from urban areas can afford it. They are also less likely to go to rural areas to work as their knowledge about the area is meagre. Hence, they end-up in settling in urban areas. Due to lower level of education in general, an overwhelming majority of professionals of health bureaucracy also come from urban areas and are also located in urban areas. Sitting in urban areas and implementing policies for rural areas might not be practical.

5.3) Lack of Institutions, Resources and Funding: Nepal is a multi-party democracy with limited number of institutions. However, there are is a lack of watchdogs who oversee these institutions. This results in low transparency about the use of resources. Though budgets are allocated, however irregularly, there are complications in using it appropriately due to complex bereaucratic system. Budgets are often being freezed because of the lack of suitable policy to implement them in a proper way. Given Nepal's low economic development and extreamly inefficient revenue collection system, the government rely on donor aids to fulfill its obligations. Donor aid on the other hand is unreliable source of income as it depends on the economic conditions of donor countries. Hence it is an unsustainable system. Additionally, Nepalese population growth is increasing in an accelerating rate and is expected to reach 30 million until 2025. The health infra-structures that exist today were built when total population was 5 million, today its 25 million.

5.4) Immigration: As other developing countries, Nepal also faces the problem of emigration. Pull factors from developed countries are attracting the Nepalese health professionals leaving a negative impact in already problematic country. Emigration to neighbouring countries like India is also high in number though it is poorly documented. Approximately 300 doctors leave Nepal for the USA and other developed countries annually (ANMC, 2008). Due to instable political situation, more and more medical students aim to leave the country after graduation. This is coupled with better opportunities for further training or post graduate studies.

2000 medical students per year, some drop-outs, 300 going abroad and the overwhelming majority staying in urban areas obviously leaves rural areas with immense scarcity of doctors. The main reasons given for not going to rural areas are as follows:

- Low Return on Investment (ROI)

- Difficult to work without medical devices in rural areas

- Lower opportunities of further training

- Difficult to manage with the employment of spouse

- Lower or no opportunity for sending the children to better quality school

- Low life standard and longer working hours

The recent introduction of compulsory rural service after graduation in Nepal has helped retain recently graduated doctors (Ghimire, 2009). Program like this are acknowledged mechanism for 13 maintaining the health workforce in underserved areas (Frehywott et al). However, the compulsory time to serve is just two years, so it might not close the gap in longer term.

5.5) Cultural Issues: In a conservative Hindu society, changing the cultural belief in order to adopt modern scientific lifestyle for better health is tremendously difficult. From the use of contraceptives till modern medicines, healthcare workers express their frustrations in convincing people to make them the use of scientific know-hows. In rural areas people trust traditional healers more than they do doctors. Additionally, there is tradition like "Chaupadi" that separates the women from house when they have mensuration. They are put in a separate house mostly outside the village completely prone to risks from wild animals, natural disasters and even drunk men. In such houses, there is normally poor hygiene which affects women's health. Other issues like sharing the same house with domestic animals, culture of prioritizing boys and not sending girls to immunize or to school, belief in spirits, as well as eating habits put more threat to the health of people.

6) Challenges of providing Healthcare during violent conflicts

6.1) Overview: Reflecting back to all the issues of providing Healthcare in the case of Nepal, it gives an impression that it is extremely difficult to launch a successful health policy so that no person should live with total absence of healthcare. In poverty stricken country like Nepal with all the issues related to bad governance, culture, lack of specialists, complex geography etc, a violent civil war worsens the condition even further. In a place where vast inequality is present, a minority of elites who live in urban areas rule over the fragile majority living in rural area and bar them from getting basic human rights including education and job opportunities, a revolution or even a civil war sooner or later is obvious. Blaikie, Cameron and Seddon's book called 'Nepal in Crisis' (1977) was one of the first prophetic alarms of the coming of the crisis in Nepal. While conducting a research in Nepal from 1974-77, they observed that the structural contradictions, stemming from 'semi-colonial experience' and 'forced stagnation in production and productivity', were pushing the country towards crisis (Basnett, 2009).

The so called "People's War" began in 1996 and lasted till 2006 and cost the lives of over 15,000 people (Douglas, 2005). Apart from this, there were other direct and indirect losses that we are going to discuss in this part.

When the Maoist violence (bombing, gun fights against governmental security personnel) increased, the government imposed a "State of Emergency"(SoE) in 2001. It had a very negative impact on Primary Health, as (Klement, Silverman, USAID) summarizes:

- Destruction of sub-health posts (as a consequence of being part of Village Development Committee (VDC) building

- Increased absence of healthcare providers at peripheral facilities

- Blockades of essential and other health commodities into certain health facilities

- Difficulties in conducting supervision and monitoring visits by regional and district-level health officers

- Disruption of the cold chain vaccines and fuel due to road blockades and power outages.

As Marco Baldan (surgeon, in ICRC) puts it "One of the first victims of war is the healthcare system itself". Sickness does not take an intermission during the time of war (Lipschultz, 2013). There will be more demand of healthcare during violent wars due to injuries, infections etc. So, the Maoist led violence was everything other than necessary.

6.2) Safety of Health Workers: "Around the world, people who risk their lives to provide health care in conflict areas are under increasing threat" (Red Cross). War ranks among the top-ten causes of death (Lopez, Murrey). Over a dozen of healthcare workers were killed and there were many cases of kidnapping, harassment, threats, prosecution by both Maoists and government sides in Nepal (Collins 2006 , Maskey 2004). The Government of Nepal (GoN) had also banned the public gathering throughout the country. Consequently, health awareness programmes could not be carried out. It also hindered the health programmes brought by NGOs.

6.3) Destruction of Infra-structures and its consequences: The motto of Maoist's so called 'People's War' was "destruction before construction" (Pettigrew et al). More than 1000 Health Posts in rural areas of Nepal were destroyed (Mukhida 2006). Destroyed roads and bridges isolated many parts of the country which directly affected the food supply which forced the remaining few people also to flee.

Consequences of such situation are high rate of mortality and worsening condition of morbidity and perhaps the complete collapse of healthcare systems. In Nepalese context nearly 200,000 people have been internally displaced (Singh 2004) and millions fled to neighbouring India. It contributed to disseminate infections like HIV, barred people from getting any health consultations and made difficult for Health planners to plan the supply of health materials and to provide appropriate care. The mass population movements created more pressure in urban areas which again caused living costs and food prices to go up. In such scenario it was difficult to do health surveillance in order to provide required vaccines for the children and to collect other healthcare related data. The USAID claims that especially in such situations, it is necessary to minimize mortality and morbidity and emergency programs must ensure the provision of adequate food, water, shelter and sanitation. Family planning services must also be made available in order to decrease maternal and child vulnerabilities.

The Maoists also forced several international agencies (important provider of Healthcare in rural areas) to leave remote western regions where help is needed the most, while the government has put several administrative roadblocks in the way of international agencies working in rural Nepal (Singh 2004). The already troubled situation was worsened by the 10 year long conflict and it pushed back the development further behind.

6.4) Reconstruction and long-term Impact: Even though Nepal had remarkable achievements in Healthcare since 1990 in-terms of maternal mortality, child mortality (Jha, Karki 2010), increase in life-expectancy and other selective primary health issues, the civil war impaired further advances. During the conflict, the budget for Healthcare and other development projects had to be diverted for security and in buying weapons to tackle the conflicts, it halted the development overall. The opportunity cost of the conflict in terms of lost output has been about 3% of Nepal's GDP (Pradhan). However, the cost of lives lost, the impact on the future of orphans, widows, deaths due to the destruction of health posts etc. are innumerable. In addition, other costs such as disruptions in trade and commerce, loss in tourism revenue, reduction in foreign investment etc. are also incalculable (Pradhan). The defence spending also curtailed spending on other sector that are crucial in Nepalese case namely education, health and infra-structural development. The atrocities committed by both Maoists and Government is still fresh in people's mind and given the current political turmoil, there is a real threat that violence can again re-escalate.

7) Conclusion: Nepal has serious health challenges from different approaches. Given its low level of economic development, the government faces precarious budget constraints for health. It is further worsened by its given culture, geography, education level etc. A ten year long civil war that occurred turned to be a disaster that placed an immense burden of re-building for the future 16

government and left hundreds of thousands of people with deteriorated health conditions. The direct and indirect costs of war have been massive. The objective of this paper was to highlight such impacts and at the same time present some challenges Nepal is facing in the process of providing Healthcare and how a violent conflict can impede further development and generate worse consequences. We come to the conclusion that the ones who are hit hard by such war are the most vulnerable people. Given the degree of impact of war, it is economically not logical to let such conflict to happen. Stakeholders should use all the resources to hinder it. Similarly, both sides should agree not to attack healthcare infrastructures or use violence against healthcare personal because they are highly important to save human lives. The case of Nepal should be used for decision making in the future regarding pre-planning prior to any possible conflicts for example in medical supplies, training of people, setting mobile clinics, vaccination and immunization programs, setting health communications, ensuring treatment to vulnerable people especially women and children etc. Lessons should also be learnt about how we can provide safety for health workers and how to install the infrastructures again in the aftermath.

References

AMERICA NEPAL MEDICAL FOUNDATION. Medical training in Nepal. (Online) 2008. Available:
http://www.anmf.net/nepal/care/training.htm (Accessed 24 March 2014)

BARRY SILVERMANN, JULIE CLEMENT, PRIMARY HEALTHCARE SERVICES IN NEPAL, Submitted for
USAID, February 2003 http://pdf.usaid.gov/pdf_docs/PNACT130.pdf (Accessed 24 March 2014)

BASNETT, Y., 2007-last update, From Politicization of Grievances to Political Violence: An Analysis
of the Maoist Movement in Nepal [Homepage of London School of Economics and Political Science],
[Online]. Available: http://www.lse.ac.uk/internationalDevelopment/publications/Working-
Papers.aspx (Accessed 22 March 2014)

COLLINS S: Assessing the health implications of Nepal's ceasefire. [http://www.thelancet.com]
Lancet 2006, 368:907 (Accessed 2 April 2014)

DIXIT, H., 2005. PRIMARY HEALTH CARE IN NEPAL. THE QUEST FOR HEALTH. . Third Edition edn.
Kathmandu, Nepal: Educational Books Publishing (P) Ltd. Kathmandu., pp. 74-97.

DIXIT, H, MARAHATTA SB, MEDICAL EDUCATION AND TRAINING IN NEPAL: SWOT ANALYSIS.
Kathmandu University Medical Journal (2008), Volume 6, Nr-3, Issue 23, 412-420.

ED DOUGLAS , National Geographic Magazine, p. 54, November 2005
FREHYWOTS, MULLAN F, PAYN PW, ROSS H. Compulsory service programmes for recruiting health
workers in remote and rural areas: do they work? Bulletin of World Health Organization 2010; 88:
364-370

GOVERNMENT OF NEPAL MINISTRY OF HEALTH AND POPULATION, 2009-last update, Fact Sheets.
Available: http://www.mohp.gov.np/english/about_moh/fact_sheet.php (Accessed 28 March 2014)

Ghimire LV. RETAINING HEALTH MANPOWER IN DEVELOPING COUNTRIES. Lancet 2009; 374: 291
INTERNATIONAL FUND FOR AGRICULTURAL DEVELOPMENT, July 2013-last update, Enabling poor
rural people to overcome poverty in Nepal. Available:
http://www.ifad.org/operations/projects/regions/pi/factsheets/nepal.pdf (Accessed 1 April 2014)

JHA, KARKI, Where is Nepal after 30 years of Alma Ata Declaration, BPKIHS, 2010, 49(178): 178-
84

KLEMENT, J. and SILVERMAN, B., 2003-last update, Primary Health Care Services in Nepal:
Program Options in Response to Conflict [Homepage of The United States Agency for International
Development], [Online]. Available: http://pdf.usaid.gov/pdf_docs/PNACT130.pdf (Accessed 2 April
2014)

LIBRARY OF CONGRESS- FEDERAL RESEARCH DIVISION, November 2005-last update, COUNTRY PROFILE: NEPAL [Homepage of Library of Congress], [Online]. Available: http://lcweb2.loc.gov/frd/cs/profiles/Nepal.pdf (Accessed 3 April 2014)

LIPSHULTZ, E., January 29,2013, 2013-last update, Securing Health Care in War Zones . Available: http://www.hcs.harvard.edu/hghr/online/securing-health-care-in-war-zones/ (Accessed 3 April 2014)

MASKEY M: Practicing politics as medicine writ large in Nepal. Development 2004, 47:122-130

MUKHIDA K: Political crisis and access to health care: A Nepalese neurosurgical experience. Bulletin of the American College of Surgeries 2006, 91:19

MURREY CJ, LOPEZ AD: Mortality by cause for eight regions of the world Global Burden of Disease Study. The Lancet 1970, 349:1269-1276

PETTIGREW J, DELFABRRO O, SHARMA M: Conflict and health in Nepal: Action for peace building. Kathmandu, DFID, GTZ & SDC 2003.

SINGH, S., 2004. Impact of long-term political conflict on population health in Nepal. CMAJ : Canadian Medical Association journal = journal de l'Association medicale canadienne, 171(12), pp. 1499-1501.

WORLD HEALTH ORGANIZATION, November 2013-last update, The right to health . Available: http://www.who.int/mediacentre/factsheets/fs323/en/ (Accessed 3 April 2014)